YEMOJA/OLOKUN

IFÁ AND THE SPIRIT OF THE OCEAN

AWO FÁ'LOKUN FATUNMBI
OMO AWO FATUNMISE, ILE IFE,
BABALAWO ÈGBÈ IFÁ, ODE REMO,
OLÚWO ILÉ ÒRÚNMÌLÁ OSHUN, OAKLAND, CA

YEMOJA / OLOKUN; Ifa and the Spirit of the Tracker
By Awo Fa'lokun Fatunmbi

© ORIGINAL PUBLICATIONS 1992

ISBN: 0-942272-33-1

Original Publications
P.O. Box 236
Old Bethpage, New York 11804-0236
(888) OCCULT-1

www.OCCULT1.com

Printed in the United States of America

ACKNOWLEDGEMENTS

The material in this book is primarily based on oral instruction from the elders of *Ifá* in Ode Remo, Ogun State, Nigeria and Ile Ife, Oshun State, Nigeria. In appreciation for their time, patience and loving concern for my training and spiritual guidance I say: *A dúpé Ègbè Ifá Ode Remo, Babalawo* Adesanya Awoyade, *Babalawo* Babalola Akinsanya, *Babalawo* Saibu Lamiyo, *Babalawo* Odujosi Awoyade, *Babalawo* Olu Taylor, *Babalawo* Abokede Arabadan, *Babalawo* Biodun Debona, *Babalawo* Oluwasina Kuti, *Babalawo* Afolabi Kuti, *Babalawo* Fagbemi Fasina, *Babalawo* Oropotoniyan and all the members of *Egbe Apetebi Ode Remo*.

Additional material in this book is based on instruction from the elders of Ile Ife, Oshun State, Nigeria. In appreciation to them I say: *A dúpé Awon Ifá Fatunmise Ègbè Ifá Ilé Ife, Jolofinpe* Falaju Fatunmise, *Babalawo* Ganiyu Olaifa Fatunmise, *Babalawo* Awoleke Awofisan Lokore, *Babalawo* Ifaioye Fatunmise, *Babalawo* Ifanimowu Fatunmise, *Babalawo* Ifasure Fatunmise, *Babalawo* Adebolu Fatunmise and all the members of *Egbe Apetebi Awon Fatunmise*.

A special thank you to the members of *Ilé Òrúnmìlà Oshun* for their continuing support and understanding: *Olori Yeye Aworo* Timi Lade, *Apetebi Orunmila, Iya l'Orisha* Oshun Miwa (Luisah Teish), *Eko'fa Iya l'Orisha* Omijinka, *Iya l'Orisha* Iya Oshun Iya Oshogbo, *Iya l'Orisha* Shango Wenwa, *Awo* Ifa Ijalagun Molu, Leona Jacobs-White, Nzinga Denny, Earthea Nance, Vance Williams, Blackberri, Salim Abdul-Jelani, Rebecca Schiros, Carol Lanigan, Zena Attig, Thisha, Rose Schadt, Xochipala Maes Valdez, Dee Orr, Nina Heft, Isoke and Earl White. A grateful thanks to *Awo* Medahochi and *Iya* Omolade.

A final thank you to Maureen Pattarelli for her work in editing this manuscript. *Orunmila a buru, a boye, a bosise.*

Awo Fá'lokun Fatunmbi
Oakland, CA

TABLE OF CONTENTS

INTRODUCTION

Yemoja/Olokun is the name of two Spiritual Forces in the West African religious tradition called *"Ifá"*. The word *Yemoja* is an elision of the Yoruba *Oriki* (praise name) *"Yeye mo oja"*, which means "Mother of Fish". The word *"Olokun"* is a contraction of *Olohun* meaning "owner", and *"okun"* meaning "Ocean". Both of these words are the names given to describe a complex convergence of Spiritual Forces that are key elements in the *Ifá* concept of fertility. Those Spiritual Forces that form the foundation of *Yemoja* and *Olokun's* role in the Spirit Realm relate to the relationship between water and birth.

According to *Ifá* cosmology the universe was created from a rock that rested on *Omi Oruṅ*, which means "Ancestral Waters". There is no literal translation for the word *Ifá*; it refers to a religious tradition, an understanding of ethics, a process of spiritual transformation and a set of scriptures that are the basis for a complex system of divination.

Ifá is found throughout the African diaspora where it spread as an integral part of Yoruba culture. The Yoruba Nation is located in the Southwestern region of Nigeria. Prior to colonization, the Yoruba Nation was a federation of city-states that were originally centered in the city of *Ilẹ́ Ifẹ̀*. According to *Ifá* myth, the Yorubas migrated to *Ilẹ́ Ifẹ̀* from the East under the leadership of a warrior chief named *Oduduwa*. It is difficult to date the time of the Yoruba move into West Africa because of limited archaeological research on the subject. Estimates range from between sixteen hundred to twenty-five hundred years ago. It is likely that migration took place over a number of generations. As the population grew, each new city-state that became a part of the Yoruba federation was governed by a chief called *"Oba"*. The position of *Oba* is a form of hereditary monarchy and each *Oba* goes through an initiation that makes them a spiritual descendant of *Oduduwa*. Traditional Yoruba political institutions are very much integrated with traditional Yoruba religious institutions. Both structures survived British rule in Nigeria, and continue to function alongside the current civil government. Within the discipline of *Ifá*, there is a body of wisdom called "*awo*", which attempts to preserve the rituals that create direct communication with Forces in Nature. *Awo* is a Yoruba word that is usually translated to mean "secret". Unfortunately, there is no real English equivalent to the word *awo*, because the word carries strong cultural and esoteric associations. In traditional Yoruba culture, *awo* refers to the hidden principles that explain the Mystery of Creation and Evolution. *Awo* is the esoteric understanding of the invisible forces that sustain dynamics and form within Nature. The essence of these invisible forces are not considered secret because they are devious, they are secret because they remain elusive, awesome in their power to transform and not readily apparent. As such they can only be grasped through direct interaction and participation. Anything which can be known by the intellect alone ceases to be *awo*.

The primal inspiration for *awo* is the communication between transcendent Spiritual Forces and human consciousness. This communication is believed to be facilitated by the Spirit of *Eṣu* who is the Divine Messenger. Working in close association with *Eṣu* is *Ogun* who, is the Spirit of Iron. *Ogun* has the power to clear away those obstacles that stand in the way of spiritual growth. According to *Ifá*, the work done by *Ogun* is guided by *Ochosi*, who as the Spirit of the Tracker has the ability to locate the shortest path to our spiritual goals. The essential goal that *Ochosi* is called upon to guide us towards is the task of building "*ìwa-pèlé*", which means "good character". This guidance takes the form of a spiritual quest which is called "*ìwakiri*". One of the functions of *Obatala* is to preserve the Mystic Vision that to those who make the quest of *ìwakiri* in search of *ìwa-pèlé*.

The function of *Yemoja* and *Olokun* are described by *Ifá* as two of many Spiritual Forces in Nature which are called "*Orisha*". The word *Orisha* means "Select Head". In a cultural context,

Orisha is a reference to the various Forces in Nature that guide consciousness. According to *Ifá*, everything in Nature has some form of consciousness called *"Orí"*. The *Orí* of all animals, plants and humans is believed to be guided by a specific Force in Nature (*Orisha*), which defines the quality of a particular form of consciousness. There are a large number of *Orisha* and each *Orisha* has its own *awo*.

The unique function of *Yemoja* and *Olokun* within the realm of *Orisha Awo* (Mysteries of Nature) is to provide the environment that sustains the continuous chain of evolution. To call an *Orisha* the Mother of Fish is to make a reference to the Source of all living creatures which exist on Earth. To call an *Orisha* the Owner of the Ocean is to make a reference to the metaphysical principle of water as one of the four primary elements of Creation. The reason that these two *Orisha* are grouped together is because they represent similar Spiritual Forces that are called by different names in different regions of West Africa. Worship of *Yemoja* is focused along the *Ogun* river, while worship of *Olokun* is prominent in Benin and Ile Ife.

Ifá teaches that all Forces in Nature come into Being through the manifestation of energy patterns called *Odu*. *Ifá* has identified and labeled 256 different *Odu* which can be thought of as different expressions of consciousness, based on the *Ifá* belief that everything which has existence has consciousness. There are *Odu* which *Ifá* describes as having the consciousness of water. This consciousness transcends the physical manifestation of hydrogen and oxygen, which are the Western scientific components of water. Water as a form of consciousness is that which flows and nurtures, it is consciousness that incubates and feeds, and it is the essence of Maternal Caring as it relates to the protection of children.

In the West these is some confusion about the role and function of *Yemoja* and *Olokun* because to some extent their role has been reversed in the diaspora. *Ifá* scripture associates *Olokun* with the Force in Nature that is called the Ocean. *Ifá* scripture associates *Yemoja* with the *Ogun* river that runs through the western region of Nigeria. However, even in Africa there is some regional variation in the understanding and interpretation of these two powerful *Orisha*. By presenting them together it is possible to shed some light on their similarities and differences.

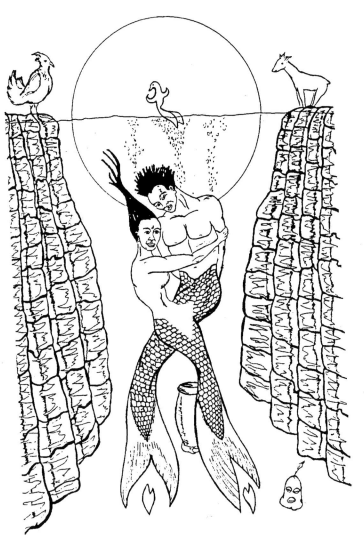

Olokun — The Owner of the Ocean

I.

ALQ IRINTÀN
YEMOJA/OLOKUN
FOLKTALES OF THE SPIRIT OF THE OCEAN

A. *YEMOJA AWO SAME* — Mother of Fish Becomes the Cloud that Produces Rain

It was *Yemoja* (The Mother of Fish) who lived alone in *Ojú Ọ̀run* (The Sky) on the day that *Olodumare* decided that *Yemoja* needed a family. *Ojú Ọ̀run* (The Sky) became *Omi Ọ̀run* (The Heavenly Waters), which gave *Yemoja* (The Mother of Fish) all the *ire* (good fortune) she needed to live and *ala* (dream). *Omi Ọ̀run* (The Ancestral Waters) was where she lived and ate, lived and ate, lived and ate until her stomach burst open creating *Ìrawọ* (the stars), *Oru* (the sun) and *irawo ti nye orun ka* (the planets).

On that day *Yemoja* came to live in *Omi aiyẹ* (Earthly Waters) where she lived and ate, lived and ate, lived and ate until her stomach burst open creating the *Orisha*. It was on that day that *Shango, Oya, Ogun, Oshun, Osanyin, Babaluaiye* and *Ibeji* came into the world.

To this day those who worship *Yemoja* say: *"Omo at'Orun gbe 'ba ajẹ ka'ri w'waiyẹ, ma ja kiki won ajẹ"*, which means, "It is the children who bring good fortune form Heaven to Earth, respect to the power of the Mothers".

Commentary: In Africa *Yemoja* is usually associated with the *Ogun River*. *Orisha* worship in the West tends to associate *Yemoja* with the Ocean; however, the Deity associated with the Ocean in

Africa is *Olokun*. This has caused some confusion regarding the role of *Yemoja* in the process of creation. In this Myth, *Yemoja* incarnates the power of fertility within all the waters of Heaven and Earth. As a principle of fertility, the African concept of *Yemoja* is associated with fresh water, salt water and heavenly water. The Idea of heavenly waters may seem highly symbolic, but it has an element of real truth. Throughout the universe the most commonly found substance is hydrogen. It forms large gas clouds in much of the space between the stars. Hydrogen is both the most abundant element in the universe and the simplest in terms of atomic structure. Water is simply the addition of oxygen to hydrogen, or H_2O. In literal terms, the abundance of hydrogen in the "heavenly waters" combined to form the stars and the planets.

The development of life on this planet was a consequence of the presence of water on the earth. Both *Ifá* and science agree that all life forms on earth evolved from the ocean. *Yemoja* as both fresh water Goddess and salt water Goddess represents the primal mother who gives birth to all living things.

B. ÒRÚNMÌLÀ IFÁ OLOKUN OSARO DAYO — The Spirit of Destiny is the Diviner of the Mystery of Abundance Found at the Bottom of the Ocean

Òrúnmìlà (the Spirit of Destiny) said goodbye to his family in *Ilé Ifẹ* on the day that he began his search for the *awo lowó* (the mystery of abundance). After a long and difficult search he discovered the *awo lowó* (the mystery of abundance) in the land that was ruled by *Olokun* (the Spirit of the Ocean). It was *Olokun* (the Spirit of the Ocean) who spent seven years giving instruction to *Òrúnmìlà* (the Spirit of Destiny) in *awo ire* (the mystery of good fortune).

Òrúnmìlà (the Spirit of Destiny) said goodbye to *Olokun* (the Spirit of the Ocean) on the day that he was preparing to return to his family in *Ilé Ifẹ*. Just before he turned to leave *Òrúnmìlà* asked *Olokun* if He had any last words of wisdom to share. *Olokun* said that there were three things that he must never do while making the journey to *Ilé Ifẹ*: he must never leave the road, he must never offer food to a stranger and he must never raise his knife in anger.

As Òrúnmìlà made his way through *igbó* (the forest), he heard an argument in the bush at the side of the road. As he approached the commotion he could hear someone calling for help. Òrúnmìlà lifted his leg to step off the path when he remembered the words of *Olokun*. Instead of helping he quickly continued on his way.

At the entrance to the next village, he told the gatekeeper about the disturbance that he had seen on the side of the road. Òrúnmìlà suggested that someone from the village should be sent back to offer assistance. The gatekeeper told Òrúnmìlà that robbers in the area used a cry for help from the bush as a trap to lure unsuspecting travelers into danger.

Òrúnmìlà found an inn near the center of the village and went inside to buy a meal. As he sat down to be served he saw an old man sitting in the center of the room. The old man had a chain around his neck that was attached to the wall. Everyone in the room seemed to ignore him as he begged for food. When a bowl of soup was placed in front of Òrúnmìlà he started to offer the old man a portion of his meal. He remembered the words of *Olokun* and decided not to share his food.

Heading back toward the path, Òrúnmìlà stopped and asked the gatekeeper about the old man who was chained to the wall of the inn. The gatekeeper told Òrúnmìlà that the old man was *Iku* (the Spirit of Death). He also told Òrúnmìlà that those who offer *Iku* food are invoking their own demise.

Òrúnmìlà entered the gates of *Ilẹ̀ Ifẹ̀* and headed directly for his compound. As he approached his house he saw his wife sitting on a stool. She was talking to a handsome young man who bent over and kissed her on the cheek. Òrúnmìlà pulled his knife from his bag and lunged towards the handsome young man. Just as he was raising the knife to attack he heard his wife say, "*A dupe omo mi*", which means "Thank you my son".

From that day on Òrúnmìlà has always praised the name of *Olokun*. Those who praise Òrúnmìlà say, "*Òrúnmìlà Ifá Olodun a-soro-dayo*", which means "The Spirit of Destiny has the

Wisdom of the Spirit of the Ocean which always provides abundance".

Commentary: This Myth is an expression of the very heart of *Ifá* belief and discipline. It is a fundamental tenet of *Ifá* that guidance from *Orisha* as it comes through divination will provide the keys for health, wealth and wisdom. In order to gain full value from this wisdom it is important to follow that guidance even when it appears to go against the inclination of a normal human response. This does not imply that *Ifá* is heartless. It does suggest that the wisdom of *Orisha* comes from a perspective that is not readily apparent to the unaided human eye.

C. ỌLỌDUMARẸ IKO — The Creator's Messenger

Olokun (the Spirit of the Ocean) consulted *Ifá* on the day that *Olokun* wanted to know if he was greater than *Ọlọdumarẹ* (the Creator). *Ifá* said that *Ọlọdumarẹ* would send a messenger to *Olokun* and that if the messenger was dressed in finer clothes than *Olokun*, it would be known who was greater in the eyes of the *Orisha* (Immortals).

On the day that *Iko* (the messenger) was to arrive, *Olokun* dressed himself in the treasures of the Sea. *Ọlọdumarẹ* sent *Agemo* (chameleon) as *Iko* (the messenger) from *Ikole Ọrun* (the Realm of the Ancestors) to *Ikole Aye* (Earth). When *Olokun* opened the door to his house, he saw *Agemo* standing in the yard wearing the same clothes that he had on. In disbelief *Olokun* closed the door and quickly changed into robes that were even more colorful. *Olokun* opened the door a second time and saw *Agemo* standing in the yard wearing the same clothes that he had changed into.

It was on that day that *Olokun* realized that he was *Olojo Oni* (the Owner of the Day) but could never be *Ọlọrun* (the Owner of the Realm of the Ancestors).

Commentary: This story is one of many *Ifá* admonitions against arrogance. The Ocean with all of its power, strength, beauty and abundance still remains dependent on the primal Forces that generated Creation itself. This story and others like it are designed as a caution for those who might become influenced by the egotism and despotism that comes with power.

II.

ÌMÒ YEMOJA/OLOKUN
THE THEOLOGICAL FUNCTION OF THE
SPIRIT OF THE OCEAN

A. YEMOJA/OLOKUN AYÀNMÓ-ÌPIN — The Spirit of the Ocean and the Concept of Destiny

The *Ifá* concept of "*àyànmó-ìpin*", which means "Destiny," is based on the belief that each person chooses their individual destiny before being born into the world. These choices materialize as those components that form human potential. Within the scope of each person's potential there exists parameters of choice that can enhance or inhibit the fullest expression of individual destiny. *Ifá* calls these possibilities "*òna ipin*", which means "road of destiny". Each decision that is made in the course of one lifetime can effect the range of possibilities that exists in the future, by either limiting or expanding the options for growth.

It is within the context of choice, or what is known in Western philosophical tradition as "free will" that *Ifá* recognizes a collection of Spiritual Forces called "*Ibora*". In Yoruba, the word *Ibora* means "Warrior". Traditionally the *Ibora* include *Eşu, Òún* and *Ochosi*. *Eşu* is the cornerstone that links the *Ibora* as they relate to the issue of spiritual growth. According to *Ifá*, each moment of existence includes a wide range of possible actions, reactions and interpretations. Those moments which require decisive action are described in *Ifá* scripture as "*òna'pade*", which means "junction in the road". Whenever a person who is trying to build character through the use of *Ifá* spiritual discipline reaches *òna'pade*, it is customary to consult *Eṣu* regarding the question of which path will bring blessings from *Orisha*.

Ifá teaches that blessings come to those who make choices that are consistent with their highest destiny. Within Yoruba culture it is understood that an individual's highest destiny is based on those choices that build "*ìwà-pèlé*", which means "good character". Those who develop good character are often described as weaving white cloth, which means creating purity and spiritual elevation in the world. The collective impact of those who weave white cloth is entering into a state of mystical union with the Chief, or the Source of White Cloth who is called "*Obatala*". This is true for everyone, even those who worship other *Orisha*. *Ifá* scripture clearly suggests what all of the *Orisha* exist as an extension of the power of consciousness that is created by the *aṣẹ* (power) of *Obatala*.

This means that all *Orisha*, including *Yemoja* and *Olokun*, exist in primal relationship to *Obatala*. This relationship is frequently ignored in *Orisha* worship as it is practiced in the West, but remains an important metaphysical principle in the *Orisha* worship of Africa. One of the primary functions of *Yemoja* and *Olokun* is to nurture physical, psychological and spiritual growth. That which is being nurtured is established by the wisdom of *Obatala* and developed through the patience and generosity of *Yemoja* and *Olokun*. It is the power of these two *Orisha* that allows for human consciousness to develop as awareness of self and world that is rooted in real experience. Because human life is imperfect, it can be chaotic, confused, painful and lonely. The *aṣẹ*, or power, of both *Yemoja* and *Olokun* is to transform traumatic experience by providing a soothing and comforting sense of the transcendent.

People throughout the world and from many different spiritual traditions go to the ocean in times of pain, sorrow and grief. It is the ability of the ocean to receive, absorb and transform these emotions into a sense of hope and joy that makes the power of *Yemoja* and *Olokun* so compelling.

B. YEMOJA/OLOKUN 'WAKIRI — The Spirit of the Ocean as the Source of Life on Earth

Ifá cosmology is based on the belief that the Primal Source of Creation is a form of Spiritual Essence called "*ạsẹ*". There is no literal translation for *ạsẹ*, although it is used in prayer to mean "May it be so".

Ifá teaches that the visible universe is generated by two dynamic forces. One is the force of "*inàlo*", which means "expansion", and the other is the force of "*isokì*", which means "contraction". The first initial manifestation of these forces is through "*imo*", which means "light", and through "*aimoyé*", which means "darkness". In *Ifá* myth, expansion and light are frequently identified with Male Spirits called "*Orisha'ko*". Contraction and darkness are frequently identified with Female Spirits called "*Orisha'bo*". Neither manifestation of *ạsẹ* is considered superior to the other and both are viewed as essential elements in the overall balance of Nature.

In *Ifá* cosmology water is a force of contraction and it is one of the primal sources of Female power. Water as a Force in Nature is constantly pressing down on itself. As you go deeper and deeper into the ocean, the pressure caused by the weight of water itself gradually changes the ecological conditions which generate life in the Sea.

It is also true that water has an expansive quality that causes streams to flow and that makes possible the process of condensation and evaporation. Because water has both qualities the Spirit of *Olokun* is understood to be androgynous. The expansive qualities of water represent the male aspect and the contractive qualities of water represent the female aspect.

Yemoja has only a female aspect and this is because she is directly related to the water which exists in the womb. The water of the womb is contractive because it creates a limited stable environment for an embryo up until the moment of birth.

Ifá cosmology teaches that there is a Great Mystery that exists at the bottom of the ocean. The bottom of the ocean is considered the sacred shrine of the ancestors and it is honored as the source of human life on Earth. In the early days of the earth's development the entire surface of the planet was covered with a liquid gas. As the earth cooled the gas solidified into land mass. While the land mass cooled the fire at the center of the earth continued to pour molten minerals into the floor of the ocean. Some Western scientists believe that life on earth emerged from the bacteria that developed from the rust that was formed as the molten minerals cooled along the bottom of the Sea.

Those first single cell life forms developed into fish, the fish developed into mammals, mammals left the ocean to live on land and eventually evolved into human life. *Olokun* was the environment in which this transformation occurred, and *Yemoja* is the principle that guided early life forms into greater levels of complexity.

Ifá teaches that everything that exists in the World has consciousness, and that the Mystery at the Bottom of the Ocean is the miracle that transformed mineral consciousness into human consciousness.

III.

ÒNA YEMOJA/OLOKUN
THE ROADS OF THE SPIRIT OF THE OCEAN

The roads of *Yemoja* are as follows:

1. *Yemoja Awoyo* — Mother of Fish, Crown of *Osumare* (the Spirit of the Rainbow) (The relationship between the Ocean and the Rainbow speaks of the blessings that come through rain.)
2. *Yemoja Okutẹ* — Mother of Fish, Who Lives in the Coastal Reef. (The coastal reef is an area of danger to boats so this aspect of *Yemoja* is considered a warrior.)
3. *Yemoja Iyaba* — The Mother of Fish as Wife of *Orunmila* (The Spirit of Destiny.)
4. *Yemoja Konla* — Mother of Fish, Who Lives in the Foam on the Surf.
5. *Yemoja Aṣẹsu* — Mother of Fish, the Messenger of *Olokun.*
6. *Yemoja Mayaleo* — Mother of Fish, the Wise Woman of the Forest (*Yemoja's* relation to the Ancestors.)
7. *Yemoja Okoto* — Mother of Fish, the Red Earth Near the Shore. (The place where sea creatures walked onto land.)
8. *Yemoja Atara Magwa Onoboyẹ* — The Mother of Fish as the Beauty of the Ocean. (The concept that the Ocean provides abundance for all those who live in the Sea.)
9. *Yemoja Yẹ'lẹ Yẹ lodo* — The Mother of Fish as the Beach and the River Bank. (The place where the water effects the ecology of the land.)
10. *Yemoja Iyaba Ti Gbẹ Ibu Omi* — Mother of Fish, Mother of *Shango* (Spirit of Lightning), Chief of the Bottom of the Water.
11. *Yemoja Yalodẹ* — Chief of the Ocean.

12. *Yemoja Afreketę* — The Mother of Fish who always walks (a reference to the constant flow of the waves against the shore.)

The roads of *Olokun* are as follows:

1. *Oba na men* — Chief of the Ocean (Male aspect of *Olokun.*)
2. *Ora* — Queen of the Ocean (in some regions of West Africa *Ora* is known as either *Mammi Watta* or *Imadese.*)
3. *Umiegho* — Wife of *Oba na men.*
4. *Igheighan* — Wife of *Oba na men.*
5. *Igbaghon* — Wife of *Oba na men.*
6. *Evbu* — Wife of *Oba na men.*

(These are some of the roads of *Olokun* as used by the *Edo* culture of Bendel State in Southern Nigeria.)

IV.

ILẸ́ ORISHA
THE SHRINE OF THE SPIRIT OF THE OCEAN

A. *ILẸ́ ORISHA ADURA* — Shrine for Prayer and Meditation to the Spirit of the Ocean

Those who are interested in honoring *Yemoja/Olokun* who have no access to either *Ifá* or *Orisha* elders can set up a shrine that may be used for meditation and prayer. The shrine can be used as a focal point for meditation that can lead to a deeper awareness, appreciation and understanding of *Yemoja* and *Olokun's* role and function within Nature. Such a shrine should be set up in a clean place and make use of either blue or red cloth as a setting for other symbolic altar pieces. In the West *Yemoja* and *Olokun* are generally associated with the color blue, representing water. However, in Africa *Olokun's* colors are red and white, which represents the principle of fertility guided by Divinity.

Almost anything collected from the ocean may be placed on the altar, such as seashells, stones, sand and even sea water will bring some of the *aṣẹ* power of the ocean to the shrine.

B. *ILẸ́ ORISHA ORIKI* — Shrine for Invocation to the Spirit of the Ocean

In the West it has become common practice to receive *Yemoja* as part of *Igbodu Orisha* (initiation), and to receive *Olokun adimu*, which means receiving *Olokun's* pot without *Igbodu* initiation. The *Ifá* calendar in Africa is based on a five day week and it is traditional for those who have received the *Igbodu* to say Oriki

Orisha (Praise Prayers) to their shrines every five days. A sample of these *Oriki* are as follows:

ORIKI YEMOJA

Ìbà Yemoja Awoyo.
I praise the Mother of Fish, Crown of the Rainbow.
Ìbà Yemoja Okutę.
I praise the Mother of Fish Who Lives in the Coastal Reef.
Ìbà Yemoja K'onla.
I praise the Mother of Fish Who Lives in the Foam on the Wave.
Yemoja a'tara magwa onoboye ba mę.
The Mother of Fish is my salvation.
Ma ja kiki won Aję.
Respect to the power of the Mothers.
Yemoja fun mi omo, a dupę.
I thank the Mother of Fish for giving me children.
Aşę.
May it be so.

ORIKI OLOKUN

Ìbà Olokun fe mi lo'rę.
I praise the Spirit of the vast and mighty Ocean.
Ìbà Olokun omo rę wa sę fun oyi o.
I praise the Spirit of the Ocean Who is beyond under-standing.
Olokun nu ni o si o ki e lu re yę toray.
Spirit of the Ocean, I will worship You as long as there is water in the Sea.
B'omi ta 'afi,
If there is peace in the Ocean,

B'ẹmi ta'afi.
> There is peace in my soul.

Olokun ni'ka lẹ,
> The Spirit of the Ocean, the ageless one,

Mo juba.
> We give respect.

Aṣẹ.
> May it be so.

C. *ADIMU YEMOJA/OLOKUN* — Offerings to the Spirit of the Ocean

In all forms of *Ifá* and *Orisha* worship it is traditional to make an offering whenever guidance or assistance is requested from Spiritual Forces. *Adimu* is a term that is generally used to refer to food and drink that is presented to the Spirit of a particular shrine. The idea behind the process of making an offering is that it would be unfair to ask for something for nothing. Those who have an unconsecrated shrine to *Yemoja/Olokun* can make the offering in their own words. Those who have a consecrated shrine to *Yemoja/ Olokun* may use the *Oriki* for *Yemoja/Olokun* when making a presentation of *Adimu*. This is usually done when a prayer requesting assistance from either *Orisha* is made. The answer to the prayer can then come through divination.

The *Adimu* for *Yemoja* is as follows:

1. Water
2. Molasses
3. Melon

The *Adimu* for *Olokun* is as follows:

1. Water
2. Molasses
3. Melon
4. Coral shells
5. Pine wood shavings

D. *EBO YEMOJA/OLOKUN* — Life Force Offerings to the Spirit of the Ocean

There is a wide range of ritual procedure in Africa involving the worship of *Orisha*. Many of the differences in ceremonial process reflect regional differences in emphasis rather than essence. The worship of *Yemoja* is strong in Abiokuta and other cities along the *Ogun* river. *Olokun* is worshiped primarily in Benin and Ile Ife. The term, "life force offering" is used in reference to the fact that many *Orisha* rituals require a preparation of a feast or communal meal. Whenever this occurs the blood from the animal that is used for the meal is given to *Orisha* as an offering. This offering is considered a reaffirmation between *Ikole Ọrun* (The Realm of the Ancestors) and *Okole Aye* (Earth). This covenant is an agreement between Spirit and humans that Spirit will provide food for the nourishment of people on earth. In return the worshipers of *Ifá* and *Orisha* agree to respect the spirit of the animal who provided the food and agree to elevate the spirit of that animal so it will return to provide food for future generations.

Whenever a life force offering is made to any of the *Orisha*, an invocation is generally made to *Ògún* as part of the process. This is a grossly misunderstood aspect of *Ifá* and *Orisha* worship which has suffered from negative stereotypes in the press and the media. It is part of *awo Ogun* (Mystery of the Spirit of Iron) to learn the inner secrets of making life force offerings. When an *Orisha* initiate is making a life force offering it should include an invocation for the *Odu Ogunda*. If the initiate is using the *Lucumí* system of *Merindinlogun*, the invocation would be to *Ogunda Meji*. In *Ifá* the invocation for life force offerings is to *Ogunda-Irẹtẹ*.

The *ebo* for *Yemoja* is as follows:

1. Hen
2. Goat

The *ebo* for *Olokun* is as follows:

1. Duck
2. Pigeon

E. *ÌWẸ YEMOJA/OLOKUN* — Cleansing for the Spirit of the Ocean

Ifá and *Orisha* make extensive use of a wide range of cleansing rituals that are designed to clear away the negative effects of illness, sorrow, grief, anger and contamination by negative spiritual influences. The most fundamental form of cleansings takes the form of invoking water. This means that the water is charged with the power of prayer to accomplish a specific purpose. Once the water has been blessed it can be used to wash specific parts of the body such as the head, the hands or the feet, or it can be used for bathing.

Those who are uninitiated may say a prayer to *Yemoja/Olokun* in their own language and breathe the prayer into the water. The healing effect of the water can be enhanced by adding salt, or by using water from the ocean.

Those who are initiated into either *Ifá* or *Orisha* may use the following prayer:

IRE OLOKUN

Irẹ ni mo nwa l'owo mi o to.
> It is good fortune that I am looking for but have not yet found.

Olokun re'lẹ Ọlọdumarẹ lo ko'rẹ wa fun mi owo ni nwa l'owo mi o to.
> Spirit of the Ocean go to the Home of the Creator and bring back the good fortune that will fulfill my Destiny.

Olugbe-rẹrẹ ko, Olugbe-rẹrẹ ko, Olugbe-rẹrẹ ko,
> The Great One Who Gives Good Things, the Great One Who Gives Good Things, the Great One Who Gives Good Things,

Gbę ręrę ko ni Olugbe-ręrę.
> Give me good things from the Great One Who Gives Things.

Olokun ba me.
> Spirit of the Ocean save us.

Nu ni o si o ki e lu re yę toray.
> We will honor you for as long as there is water in the Ocean.

Olokun fę mi lo'rę, mo dupę.
> Spirit of the Endless Bottomless Ocean, we thank you.

Aşę.
> May it be so.

IRE YEMOJA

Ìbà şę Yemoja Ibikeji odo.
> I respect the Spirit of the Mother of Fish, the Goddess of the Sea.

Omo at'Orun 'gbę 'gba aję ka'ri w'aiyę.
> It is children who bring good fortune from the Realm of the Ancestors to Earth.

Yemoja at'Orun 'gbę 'gba omo ka'ri w'aiyę.
> It is the Mother of Fish who brings children from the Realm of the Ancestors to Earth.

Yemoja fun me la l'afia, mo dupę.
> Mother of Fish bring us good health, we thank you.

Yemoja nuaa jeke awon o'iku.
> Mother of Fish protect us from sickness and death.

Ma ja kiki wa Òrun.
> We praise the power of the Realm of the Ancestors.

B'omi ta 'afi a row pon aşę Yemoja.
> May there be peace in the waters that bring the power of the Spirit of the Mother of Fish.

Aşę.
> May it be so.

V.

ORISHA 'GUN
THE SPIRIT OF THE OCEAN AND THE
MEANING OF SPIRIT POSSESSION

Those who practice the religion of *Ifá* in Africa are generally members of a society that worships a single *Orisha*. These societies are usually referred to by the term "*ẹgbẹ̀*", which means "heart", as in the expression "the heart of the matter". Those who worship *Yemoja* would be members of *Ẹgbẹ̀ Yemoja*, and those who worship *Olokun* would be members of *Ẹgbẹ̀ Olokun*. In Abiokuta the worship of *Yemoja* is closely associated with the worship of *Ògún* (The Spirit of Iron), and in Benin the worship of *Olokun* is closely associated with *Shango* (The Spirit of Lightning).

Each *Ẹgbẹ̀ Orisha* preserves the oral history, myth and wisdom associated with *Awo Orisha* (The Mystery as particular Force in Nature). Part of the wisdom that is preserved concerns the discipline used to access altered states of consciousness. Western literature on *Orisha* tends to refer to these states as "possession". This term is inadequate to describe the various forms of trance that are used to assist the *Orisha* worshiper in their understanding of the Mysteries of Being.

Ifá teaches that it is possible to access both *Orisha* (Forces in Nature) and *Egun* (ancestors) through the disciplined use of dreams. The word "*ala*" is used in Yoruba to mean "dream". *Ala* is the last part of the word *Obatala* (The Spirit of the Chief of White Cloth), and it suggests that the dream state is closely associated with the source of consciousness itself. The word "*alala*" is the word for "dreamer". Because dreamer has a positive connotation in *Ifá*, the word *alala* is a reference to those who are able to make effective use of dreams. *Alala* appears to be a contraction of *ala* and *ala*. In Yoruba words are often repeated for emphasis or to establish relative relationships. To use the word *ala* twice suggests that the reference to dreamer is an expression of the belief that dreams can access the true source of inner thoughts.

Ifá teaches that it is possible to develop an ongoing relationship with *Orisha* that makes a person sensitive to the influence of *Orisha* on a daily basis that effects their immediate environment. In English this is usually referred to as a highly developed intuition. The Yoruba word for intuition is *"ogbon inu"*, which translates literally to mean "the stomach of the earth". *Ifá* metaphysics is based on the idea that those Forces in Nature that sustain life on earth establish certain guidelines for living in harmony with Creation. The development of a sensitivity to these forces is part of the discipline of *Orisha* worship and this sensitivity is called *"ogbon inu"*.

There are a number of words that are used to describe those altered states that are commonly referred to as possession. In conjunction with *Orisha* the word *"jogun"*, meaning either "I possess", or "I have" is used to describe a close spiritual connection with Spirit. The phrase *"Orisha' gun"*, is used to describe those who have assumed the characteristics of a particular *Orisha*.

The more common term for possession is *"iní"*. This word reveals the *Ifá* perspective on those trance states which represent a deep connection with the *aṣẹ* (power) of *Orisha*. The word *iní* appears to be a contraction of *"i"*, which is a personal pronoun, and *"ni"* which is the verb "to be". To use the phrase "I am" as a reference to possession suggests that what is frequently thought of as an intrusion from outside forces is more accurately understood as a process of unlocking the *awo* (mystery) of the inner self. *Ifá* teaches that every person comes to Earth with a spark of divinity at the foundation of their *orí* (inner spirit). Part of the discipline of *Orisha* worship is to access this spark of divinity. This is generally accomplished through initiation, which is designed to guide the initiate towards access to the inner self, which in turn forms a transcendent link to *Orisha*, which is closest to the consciousness of the initiate.

Those who have been through initiation for either *Yemoja* or *Olokun* can enhance their access to *ini* at the same time that offerings are made to their shrine on a five day cycle. This is done by saying *Oriki* in front of the initiate's *Orisha* shrine. When the *Oriki* is spoken a candle is lit near the *Orisha* pot and a glass of water is placed near the candle. After the *Oriki* has been completed, the initiate breathes into the glass of water and says the word "*to*", which means "enough". The word *to* is used at the end of *Oriki* as a seal or lock to attach the invocation to whatever it is spoken on to.

Using the index finger, the ring finger and the little finger on the left hand, the initiate dips the fingers in the water and runs the water from between the forehead across the top of the head and down the back of the neck. When the fingers are between the eyebrows say, "*iwaju*", which is the name of the power center at the forehead. When the fingers are on the top of the head say, "*ori*", which is the name of the power center at the crown of the skull. When the fingers are on the back of the neck say, "*ipako*", which is the name of the power center at the base of the skull.

A sample of the type of *Oriki* that is used for this process is as follows:

ORIKI OLOKUN

Ìbà Olokun,
    I respect the Spirit of the Ocean,
Ìbà 'ge Olojo Oni.
    I respect the Owner of the Day.
Olokun pęlę o.
    Spirit of the Ocean, I greet you.
Olokun pęlę o.
    Spirit of the Ocean, I greet you.
Olokun pęlę o.
    Spirit of the Ocean, I greet you.
Ni igba meta.
    I greet You three times.
Olokun nu ni o se o ki e lu re ye toray.
    Spirit of the Ocean, I will worship You for as long as
    there is water in the Sea.

B'omi ta 'afi.
> Let there be peace in the water.

B'ẹmí ta 'afi.
> Let there be peace in my soul.

Mo juba.
> I give praise.

Aṣẹ.
> May it be so.

ORIKI YEMOJA

Ìbà Yemoja Yalode.
> I respect the Mother of Fish the Queen of the Sea.

Agbẹ ni igbẹ 're ki Yemoja Ibikeji odo.
> It is the bird who delivers abundance to the Mother of Fish, Goddess of the Sea.

Yemoja pẹlẹ o.
> Mother of Fish I greet You.

Yemoja pẹlẹ o.
> Mother of Fish I greet You.

Yemoja pẹlẹ o.
> Mother of Fish I greet You.

Ni igba meta.
> I greet You three times.

Yemoja ni 'ka lẹ,
> Mother of Fish, the Ageless One,

Oro ti ase fun Yemoja ni awon omo re wa sẹ fun oyi o.
> The power of transformation that comes from the Mother of Fish is beyond understanding.

Yemoja ba me.
> Mother of Fish save me.

A juba.
> I give praise.

Aṣẹ.
> May it be so.

VI.

ORIN YEMOJA/OLOKUN
SONG FOR THE SPIRIT OF THE OCEAN

YEMOJA

Call: *Yemoja e olodo awoye Yemoja.*
(Mother of Fish, Chief of Woman's Mysteries, Mother of Fish).
Response: Repeat.
Call: *Yemoja kole Yemoja lara mi.*
(Mother of Fish enter my body).
Response: Repeat.
Call: *Yemoja Orisha Orisha Yemoja fun mi lowo.*
(Mother of Fish, Spirit, Spirit, Mother of Fish give me abundance).
Response: *Yemoja Orisha Orisha Yemoja.*
(Mother of Fish, Spirit, Spirit, Mother of Fish).
Call: *Fun mi lowo.*
(Give me abundance).
Response: *Wami odara odara wami Yemoja fun mi lowo.*
(Bring me good things, good things, Mother of Fish bring me abundance).
Call: *Yemoja fun mi lowo.*
(Mother of Fish bring me abundance).
Response: *Wami odara odara wami.*
(Bring me good things, good things, bring me).

Call: *Yemoja asesu asesu Yemoja.* (2 times).
(Mother of Fish, mouth of power, mouth of power, Mother of Fish).

Yemoja olodo olodo Yemoja. (2 times)
    (Mother of Fish Queen, Queen Mother of Fish).
Response: Repeat
Call: *Yemoja olodo olodo Yemoja.* *(2 times)*
    (Mother of Fish Queen, Queen Mother of Fish).
Response: Repeat

ORIN OLOKUN

Call: *Olokun ba wa o.*
    (Spirit of the Ocean save us).
Response: *Ba wa Orisha ba wo o oe.*
    (Save us Spirit save us al).

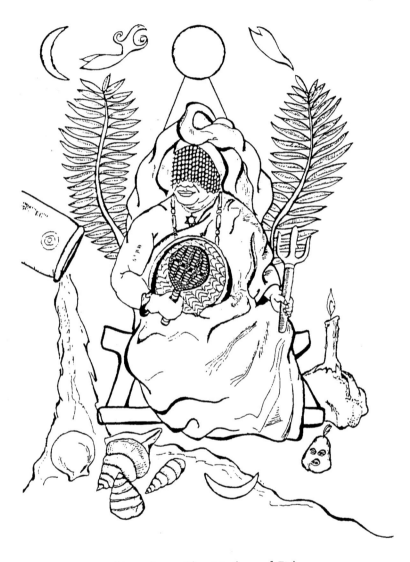

Yemoja — The Mother of Fish

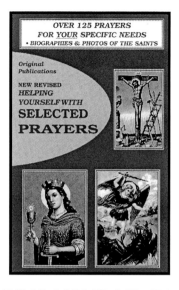

ITEM #214
$8.95

HELPING YOURSELF WITH SELECTED PRAYERS

NOW OVER 130,000 IN PRINT!

The New Revised Helping Yourself with Selected Prayers provides an English translation for over 125 prayers of various religious beliefs. These prayers will provide a foundation upon which you can build your faith and beliefs. It is through this faith that your prayers will be fulfilled.

An index is provided to help the reader find the appropriate prayer for his or her particular request. The index also includes suggestions regarding the appropriate candle to burn while saying a particular prayer.

The devotions within these pages will help you pray consciously, vigorously, sincerely and honestly. True prayer can only come from within yourself.

ISBN 0-942272-01-3 5½"x 8½" 112 pages $8.95

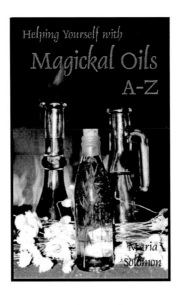

ITEM #172
$9.95

HELPING YOURSELF WITH
MAGICKAL OILS A-Z

BY MARIA SOLOMON

The most thorough and comprehensive
workbook available on the

Magickal Powers of
Over 1000 Oils!

Easy to follow step-by-step instructions
for more than 1500
Spells, Recipes and Rituals for
Love, Money, Luck, Protection
and much more!

ISBN 0-942272-49-8 5½"x 8½" $9.95

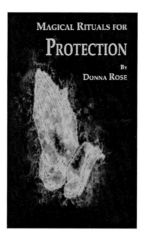

MAGICAL RITUALS FOR
PROTECTION
by Donna Rose

Oils, Incense & Powders for Protection
Magical Herbs for Protection
Magical Gemstones for Protection
Psalms for Protection
Prayers for Protection

Magical Spells for Protection

Cleansing Ritual
Purification Spell to Cleanse Yourself
Repelling Negativity
To Annul an Evil Spell
Defeat an Enemy's Evil
Binding Someone Annoying Spell
Reversing Spell to Send Back a Curse or Hex
Dragons Blood Reed Spell To Lift Hexes and Jinxes
Overcome an Enemy
Cast Off The Influence Of The Evil Eye
Spell Against Hoodoos Haunts and Evil Works
Spell to Make Someone Move Away

ORIGINAL PUBLICATIONS / www.OCCULT1.com

- ☐ **HELPING YOURSELF WITH SELECTED PRAYERS;** *Volume 1*; $8.95
- ☐ **HELPING YOURSELF WITH SELECTED PRAYERS:** *Volume 2*; $9.95
- ☐ **MASTER BOOK OF CANDLE BURNING WITH PSALMS;** $9.95
- ☐ **COMPLETE BOOK OF BATHS:** Robert Laremy - $9.95
- ☐ **UNHEXING AND JINX REMOVING;** by Donna Rose - $6.95
- ☐ **SUCCESS AND POWER THROUGH PSALMS;** by Donna Rose - $6.95
- ☐ **MAGICAL RITUALS FOR MONEY;** by Donna Rose - $7.95
- ☐ **MAGICAL RITUALS FOR LOVE;** by Donna Rose - $7.95
- ☐ **MAGICAL RITUALS FOR PROTECTION;** by Donna Rose - $7.95
- ☐ **PSALM WORKBOOK:** Robert Laremy - $11.95
- ☐ **SPIRITUAL CLEANSINGS & PSYCHIC PROTECTION;** Robert Laremy $9.95
- ☐ **NEW REVISED MASTER BOOK OF CANDLEBURNING;** Gamache - $9.95
- ☐ **THE MAGIC CANDLE;** Charmaine Dey $8.95
- ☐ **NEW REV. 6&7 BKS. OF MOSES;** Wippler $14.95
- ☐ **MYSTERY OF THE LONG LOST 8,9,10TH BOOKS OF MOSES;** Gamache - $9.95
- ☐ **VOODOO & HOODOO;** by Jim Haskins - $16.95
- ☐ **COMPLETE BOOK OF VOODOO:** Robert Pelton $16.95
- ☐ **PAPA JIM'S HERBAL MAGIC WORKBOOK;** Papa Jim - $9.95
- ☐ **HELPING YOURSELF WITH MAGICAL OILS A-Z;** Maria Solomon - $11.95
- ☐ **SANTERIA FORMULARY & SPELLBOOK;** Carlos Montenegro - $16.95
- ☐ **READING YOUR FUTURE IN THE CARDS;** Eden - $7.95
- ☐ **SANTERIA; AFRICAN MAGIC IN LATIN AMERICA;** Wippler $14.95
- ☐ **SANTERIA EXERIENCE;** Wippler $14.95
- ☐ **POWERS OF THE ORISHAS;** Wippler $9.95
- ☐ **THE BOOK ON PALO;** Raul Canizares $21.95
- ☐ **ESHU ELLEGGUA; IFA and the Divine Messenger;** Fatunmbi $7.95
- ☐ **SHANGO; IFA and the Spirit of Lightning;** $7.95
- ☐ **BABALU AYE; Santeria and the Lord of Pestilence;** Canizares $7.95
- ☐ **OSHUN: IFA and the Spirit of the River;** Fatunmbi $7.95
- ☐ **OGUN: IFA and the Spirit of Iron;** Fatunmbi $7.95
- ☐ **OYA: IFA and the Spirit of the Wind;** Fatunmbi $7.95
- ☐ **YEMOJA / OLOKUN: IFA and the Spirit of the Ocean;** Fatunmbi $7.95
- ☐ **ORUNLA: Santeria and the Orisha of Divination;** Canizares $6.95
- ☐ **OSANYIN: Santeria and the Orisha of Lord of Plants;** Canizares $6.95
- ☐ **OBATALA: IFA and the Spirit of the White Cloth;** Fatunmbi $7.95
- ☐ **OCHOSI: IFA and the Spirit of the Tracker;** Fatunmbi $7.95
- ☐ **AGANJU: Santeria and the Orisha Volcanoes & Wilderness** $6.95

NAME _____ TELEPHONE _____

ADDRESS _____

CITY _____ STATE _____ ZIP _____

Visa / Mastercard / Discover
American Express   **TOLL FREE (888) 622-8581 -OR- (516) 605-0547**

TO ORDER BY MAIL: CHECK THE BOXES NEXT TO YOUR SELECTIONS. ADD THE TOTAL. SHIPPING COSTS ARE $3.50 FOR THE FIRST BOOK PLUS 75 CENTS FOR EACH ADDITIONAL BOOK. NEW YORK STATE RESIDENTS PLEASE ADD 8.25% SALES TAX. ALL ORDERS SHIP IN 14 DAYS. SORRY, NO C.O.D.'S. SEND ORDERS TO THE ADDRESS BELOW.

ORIGINAL PUBLICATIONS • P.O. BOX 236, OLD BETHPAGE, NY 11804-0236

TOLL FREE: 1(888) OCCULT-1   **WWW.OCCULT1.COM**